EASY BREAKFAST IDEAS FOR WEIGHT LOSS

Effortless Ways To Shed Pounds With Nutritious Recipes

By

NORMAN FIELDS

TABLE OF CONTENT

INTRODUCTION

HOW BREAKFAST CAN HELP YOU LOSE WEIGHT

As the sun gently rises, casting a golden hue across the morning sky, there exists a transformative ritual often overlooked in our fast-paced lives: breakfast. Beyond its role in satiating hunger, breakfast holds profound implications for our health and well-being, particularly in the realm of weight management. Imagine this: a morning ritual that not only fuels your body but sets a foundation for sustained energy and balanced nutrition throughout the day.

Consider the story of Mark, a father juggling the demands of career and family. For years, Mark skipped breakfast or hastily grabbed something on the go, unaware of its impact on his health. When he began incorporating wholesome breakfasts into his routine, he noticed a significant change. His cravings stabilized, his energy levels improved, and he found it easier to maintain a healthy weight. What started as a simple adjustment blossomed into a newfound appreciation for the role of breakfast in overall well-being.

This book is a practical guide designed to illuminate the benefits of a well-rounded breakfast, specifically tailored to support weight loss goals. It's about embracing the potential of each morning as an opportunity to nourish and energize your body. Through easy-to-follow recipes and insightful tips, you'll discover how simple adjustments in your morning routine can yield profound results in your health journey.

CHAPTER 1

QUICK AND NUTRITIOUS SMOOTHIES

Smoothies are not just a morning treat; they are a powerful tool in your journey towards weight loss. These blended beverages offer a convenient way to pack essential nutrients into one delicious drink, perfect for busy mornings or as a refreshing snack. Here, we delve into a collection of smoothie recipes designed to nourish your body while supporting your weight loss goals.

1.GREEN GODDESS SMOOTHIE

- **Ingredients**:
  - Spinach
  - Cucumber
  - Banana
  - Greek yogurt
  - Almond Milk

- **Preparation**:
  - Blend spinach, cucumber, banana, Greek yogurt, and almond milk until smooth.
  - Serve chilled.

- **Health Benefits**:

Spinach and cucumber are low in calories and high in fiber, aiding in digestion and keeping you full longer. Greek yogurt provides protein, which is essential for muscle maintenance and satiety. Bananas add natural sweetness and potassium, which helps regulate blood pressure.

2. BERRY BLAST SMOOTHIE

- **Ingredients**:
  - Mixed berries (strawberries, blueberries, raspberries)
  - Spinach
  - Chia Seeds
  - Coconut Water

- **Preparation**:
  - Blend mixed berries, spinach, chia seeds, and coconut water until smooth.
  - Enjoy immediately.

- **Health Benefits**:
Berries are rich in antioxidants, which combat inflammation and support heart health. Chia seeds

are high in omega-3 fatty acids, which promote brain health and reduce inflammation. Coconut water is hydrating and provides electrolytes, making it an excellent post-workout drink.

3. TROPICAL PARADISE SMOOTHIE

- **Ingredients**:
  - Pineapple
  - Mango
  - Banana
  - Coconut Milk
  - Greek Yogurt

- **Preparation**:
  - Blend pineapple, mango, banana, coconut milk, and Greek yogurt until creamy.
  - Garnish with shredded coconut if desired.

- **Health Benefits**:

Pineapple and mango are packed with vitamins C and A, which boost the immune system and improve skin health. Coconut milk contains healthy fats that can help you feel satiated. Greek yogurt adds protein, aiding in muscle repair and maintenance.

4. PROTEIN POWER SMOOTHIE

- Ingredients:
- Almond butter
- Banana
- Spinach
- Almond milk
- Protein powder (optional).

- Preparation:
- Blend almond butter, banana, spinach, almond milk, and protein powder (if using) until well combined.
- Serve cold.

- **Health Benefits**:

Almond butter provides healthy fats and protein, which help stabilize blood sugar levels and keep you feeling full. Spinach offers iron and other essential nutrients. Adding protein powder can further boost the protein content, supporting muscle growth and recovery.

5. AVOCADO DELIGHT SMOOTHIE

- Ingredients:
- Avocado
- Spinach
- Cucumber
- Lemon Juice
- Honey (optional),
- Water

- Preparation:
- Blend avocado, spinach, cucumber, lemon juice, honey (if using), and water until smooth.
- Adjust sweetness to taste.

- Health Benefits:

Avocado is rich in monounsaturated fats, which are good for heart health and help keep you satisfied. Spinach and cucumber add fiber and hydration. Lemon juice provides a refreshing taste and is high in vitamin C, which supports the immune system.

Each smoothie is carefully crafted to provide a balance of nutrients, including fiber, protein, and vitamins, to keep you feeling full and energized. Incorporating these smoothies into your breakfast routine can help curb cravings, support digestion, and promote overall wellness.

CHAPTER 2

ENERGIZING EGG RECIPES

Eggs are a versatile and protein-rich food that can be a cornerstone of a healthy breakfast. They provide sustained energy, keeping you full and focused throughout the morning. This chapter features a variety of egg-based recipes that are both delicious and supportive of your weight loss goals.

1. SPINACH AND FETA OMELET

- **Ingredients**:
  - 2 eggs
  - Handful Of Fresh Spinach
  - 1/4 Cup Crumbled Feta Cheese
  - Salt and Pepper to taste
  - Olive Oil

- **Preparation**:
  - Beat the eggs in a bowl and season with salt and pepper. In a nonstick pan, warm the olive oil over medium heat.
  - Add spinach and cook until wilted.

- The beaten eggs should be added and cooked until set.
- Sprinkle feta cheese on top
- fold the omelet, and serve hot.

- Health Benefits:

Eggs provide high-quality protein, which is vital for muscle repair and satiety. Spinach adds fiber, iron, and vitamins, while feta cheese contributes calcium and a burst of flavor.

2. VEGGIE-PACKED SCRAMBLE

- **Ingredients**:
  - 3 eggs
  - 1/4 cup diced bell peppers
  - 1/4 cup diced tomatoes
  - 1/4 cup chopped onions
  - 1/4 cup chopped mushrooms
  - Salt and pepper to taste
  - Olive oil.

- **Preparation**:
  - Beat the eggs in a bowl and season with salt and pepper.
  - Apply heat to the olive oil in a pan using a medium-high flame.

- Add bell peppers, tomatoes, onions, and mushrooms, and sauté until tender.
- Add the whisked eggs and stir until fully cooked.
- Serve warm.

- Health Benefits:
This scramble is packed with vegetables that provide fiber, vitamins, and antioxidants. Eggs add protein to keep you feeling satisfied longer.

3. AVOCADO EGG SALAD

- Ingredients:
- 2 hard-boiled egg
- 1 ripe avocado
- 1 tablespoon Greek yogurt
- 1 teaspoon lemon juice
- Salt and pepper to taste.

- Preparation:
- Peel and chop the hard-boiled eggs.
- In a bowl, mash the avocado and mix with Greek yogurt, lemon juice, salt, and pepper.
- Add the chopped eggs and stir until thoroughly mixed.

- Serve on whole-grain toast or as a dip with fresh vegetables.

- Health Benefits:
Avocado provides healthy fats and fiber, while eggs add protein. Greek yogurt adds creaminess and additional protein, making this salad both nutritious and satisfying.

4. EGG AND VEGETABLE MUFFINS

- **Ingredients**:
  - 6 eggs
  - 1/2 cup diced bell peppers
  - 1/2 cup chopped spinach
  - 1/4 cup diced onions
  - Salt and pepper to taste
  - Olive oil.

- **Preparation**:
  - Preheat the oven to 375°F (190°C).
  - Beat the eggs and add salt and pepper to taste in a bowl.
  - Grease a muffin tin with olive oil.

- Divide the bell peppers, spinach, and onions evenly among the muffin cups.
- Pour the beaten eggs over the vegetables.
- Bake the eggs for twenty to twenty-five minutes, or until they set.
- Let cool slightly before serving.

- Health Benefits:

These muffins are an excellent way to incorporate vegetables into your breakfast. They are portable and convenient for busy mornings, providing protein, fiber, and essential vitamins.

5. POACHED EGGS WITH ASPARAGUS

- **Ingredients**:
  - 2 eggs
  - 1 bunch of asparagus
  - 1 tablespoon white vinegar
  - Salt and pepper to taste
  - Olive oil.

- **Preparation**:
  - Bring a pot of water to a simmer and add the vinegar.
  - Crack the eggs into separate cups.
  - Gently slide the eggs into the water and poach for 3-4 minutes until the whites are

set but the yolks are still runny.

- Meanwhile, heat olive oil in a pan and sauté the asparagus until tender.
- Season with salt and pepper.
- Serve the poached eggs over the asparagus.

- Health Benefits:
Poached eggs are a low-calorie way to enjoy eggs, and asparagus is a great source of fiber, folate, and vitamins A, C, and K. This dish is light yet satisfying, perfect for a healthy breakfast.

Eggs are a nutritional powerhouse, offering protein, healthy fats, and a variety of vitamins and minerals. Incorporating these recipes into your morning routine can provide sustained energy and help you stay on track with your weight loss goals.

CHAPTER 3

LOW-CARB BREAKFAST IDEAS

Starting your day with a low-carb breakfast can help manage hunger and keep energy levels stable. This chapter presents a variety of satisfying and nutrient-dense recipes designed to support your weight loss journey.

1. CAULIFLOWER HASH BROWNS

- **Ingredients**:
  - 1 head of cauliflower
  - 1 egg
  - 1/4 cup grated Parmesan cheese
  - Salt and pepper to taste
  - Olive oil.

- **Preparation**:
  - Grate the cauliflower and microwave it for about 5 minutes.
  - Allow it to cool, then squeeze out excess water using a clean cloth.

- In a bowl, mix the cauliflower, egg, cheese, salt, and pepper.
- Form the mixture into small patties.
- Heat olive oil in a skillet over medium heat and cook the patties until they are golden brown on both sides.
- Serve warm.

- Health Benefits:

Cauliflower provides fiber and essential vitamins while being low in carbs. The egg and cheese add protein and healthy fats, making this a balanced and nutritious start to your day.

2. AVOCADO AND EGG BREAKFAST BOWL

- **Ingredients**:
  - 1 avocado
  - 2 eggs
  - 1/4 cup cherry tomatoes
  - Salt and pepper to taste
  - Olive oil.

-**Preparation**:
  - Divide the avocado into two halves and extract the pit.
  - Remove the inner part and crush it in a container.
  - Cook the eggs to your preference (boiled, poached, or scrambled).

- Place the mashed avocado in a bowl and top with the eggs and cherry tomatoes.
- Apply a layer of olive oil and season with salt and pepper.
- Enjoy immediately.

- Health Benefits:

Avocados are rich in healthy fats and fiber, which help keep you full. Eggs provide high-quality protein, and cherry tomatoes add antioxidants and vitamins.

3. GREEK YOGURT AND NUT PARFAIT

- **Ingredients**:
  - 1 cup Greek yogurt
  - 1/4 cup chopped nuts (such as almonds or walnuts)
  - 1 tablespoon chia seeds
  - A few drops of vanilla extract.

- **Preparation**:
  - In a glass or bowl, layer Greek yogurt with chopped nuts and chia seeds.
  - Incorporate a small amount of vanilla extract to enhance the taste.
  - Serve chilled.

- **Health Benefits**:

Greek yogurt is packed with protein and probiotics, supporting digestive health. Nuts add healthy fats and protein, while chia seeds provide fiber and omega-3 fatty acids.

4. SMOKED SALMON AND AVOCADO PLATE

- **Ingredients**:
  - 1 avocado,
  - 3 oz smoked salmon
  - 1 tablespoon capers
  - A squeeze of lemon juice,
  - Salt and pepper to taste.

- **Preparation**:
  - Slice the avocado and arrange it on a plate.
  - Add the smoked salmon and sprinkle with capers.
  - Drizzle lemon juice over the top and season with salt and pepper.
  - Serve immediately.

- **Health Benefits**:

Smoked salmon offers omega-3 fatty acids and protein, beneficial for heart health. Avocado contributes healthy fats and fiber, making this dish both nourishing and satisfying.

5. ZUCCHINI AND CHEESE OMELET

- **Ingredients**:
- 3 eggs
- 1 small zucchini (thinly sliced)
- 1/4 cup grated cheese
- Salt and pepper to taste
- Olive oil.

- **Preparation**:
- Beat the eggs in a bowl and season with salt and pepper.
- Warm the olive oil in a non-stick skillet on medium heat.
- Add the zucchini slices and cook until they soften.

- Pour the beaten eggs over the zucchini and cook until the eggs are almost set.
- Disperse the cheese evenly over the surface and then fold the omelet in half.
- Cook until the cheese melts.
- Serve hot.

- **Health Benefits**:
Zucchini is low in carbohydrates and high in vitamins and minerals. Eggs offer protein and healthy fats, and cheese adds calcium and additional protein, making this a well-rounded low-carb breakfast.

Low-carb breakfasts can help control cravings and maintain

energy throughout the day. Including these recipes in your morning routine can lead to both satisfying and nutritious meals that support your weight loss efforts.

CHAPTER 4

SIMPLE OATMEAL VARIATIONS

Oatmeal is a versatile and nutritious breakfast option that can be customized to suit your taste while supporting weight loss. This chapter presents a variety of oatmeal recipes that are easy to prepare and packed with nutrients to fuel your morning.

1. BERRY AND ALMOND OATMEAL

- Ingredients:
  - 1/2 cup rolled oats
  - 1 cup almond milk
  - 1/2 cup mixed berries
  - 1 tablespoon sliced almonds
  - 1 teaspoon honey.

- **Preparation**:
  - In a saucepan combine oats and almond milk.
  - Bring to a boil, then reduce heat and simmer for about 5 minutes until the oats are tender.
  - Stir in the berries and cook for another minute.

- Transfer to a bowl and top with sliced almonds and a drizzle of honey.
- Serve warm.

- Health Benefits:
Oats provide fiber, which helps with digestion and keeps you feeling full. Berries add antioxidants and vitamins, while almonds contribute healthy fats and protein.

2. APPLE CINNAMON OATMEAL

- **Ingredients**:
  - 1/2 cup rolled oats
  - 1 cup water or milk
  - 1 small apple (chopped)
  - 1/2 teaspoon cinnamon
  - 1 teaspoon maple syrup.

- **Preparation**:
  - Combine oats, water or milk, chopped apple, and cinnamon in a saucepan.
  - Bring to a boil, then reduce heat and simmer for about 5 minutes until the oats are cooked and the apple is tender.

- Stir in the maple syrup.
- Serve warm.

- Health Benefits:
Apples are an excellent source of both fiber and vitamin C. Cinnamon can help regulate blood sugar levels, and oats provide long-lasting energy and satiety.

3. PEANUT BUTTER BANANA OATMEAL

- **Ingredients**:
  - 1/2 cup rolled oats
  - 1 cup milk
  - 1 tablespoon peanut butter
  - 1 small banana (sliced)
  - A pinch of salt.

- **Preparation**:
  - In a saucepan, cook the oats and milk over medium heat until the oats are tender.
  - Stir in the peanut butter and salt.
  - Spoon into a bowl and garnish with banana slices.
  - Serve warm.

- **Health Benefits**:
Peanut butter adds protein and healthy fats, which help keep you full longer. Bananas provide potassium and natural sweetness, making this a balanced and satisfying breakfast.

4. CHOCOLATE CHIA OATMEAL

- Ingredients:

1/2 cup rolled oats

1 cup almond milk

1 tablespoon chia seeds

1 tablespoon cocoa powder

1 teaspoon honey.

- Preparation:

- Combine oats, almond milk, chia seeds, and cocoa powder in a saucepan.
- Bring to a boil, then reduce heat and simmer for about 5 minutes until the oats are tender and the mixture thickens.

- Stir in the honey.
- Serve warm.

- Health Benefits:
Chia seeds are a great source of fiber and omega-3 fatty acids. Cocoa powder provides antioxidants, and oats offer a hearty, fiber-rich base.

5. SAVORY SPINACH AND EGG OATMEAL

- **Ingredients**:
  - 1/2 cup rolled oats
  - 1 cup water
  - 1 cup fresh spinach (chopped)
  - 1 egg
  - Salt and pepper to taste
  - Olive oil.

- **Preparation**:
  - In a saucepan, cook the oats and water over medium heat until the oats are tender.
  - Add the chopped spinach and cook, stirring, until it wilts.

- In a separate skillet, cook the egg to your liking (fried or poached).
- Transfer the oatmeal to a bowl, top with the egg, and season with salt and pepper.
- Drizzle with olive oil.
- Serve warm.

- **Health Benefits**:
Spinach is rich in vitamins and minerals, and eggs provide protein to help keep you full. This savory oatmeal is a nutrient-dense way to start your day.

Oatmeal is a versatile base that can be adapted to various flavors and ingredients, making it an excellent option for a healthy breakfast. These simple variations provide a mix of nutrients to support your weight loss goals and keep you energized throughout the morning.

CHAPTER 5

EASY TOAST AND SANDWICH COMBOS

Toast and sandwiches offer quick and versatile breakfast options. This chapter introduces a variety of recipes that are easy to prepare, nutritious, and perfect for starting your day on the right foot.

1. AVOCADO AND TOMATO TOAST

- **Ingredients**:
  - 1 slice of whole-grain bread
  - 1/2 avocado
  - 1/4 cup cherry tomatoes (halved)
  - Salt and pepper to taste
  - lemon juice.

- **Preparation**:
  - Toast the bread to your desired crispiness.
  - Once the avocado has been mashed, spread it out onto the toast.

- Top with cherry tomatoes, a squeeze of lemon juice, and season with salt and pepper.
- Serve immediately.

- **Health Benefits**:

Avocado provides healthy fats and fiber, while tomatoes add antioxidants and vitamins. Bread made from whole grains is a better source of nutrients and fiber.

2. PEANUT BUTTER AND BANANA SANDWICH

- **Ingredients**:
  - 2 slices of whole-grain bread
  - 2 tablespoons of peanut butter
  - 1 small banana (sliced).

- **Preparation**:
  - Spread peanut butter on one slice of bread.
  - Arrange banana slices on top and cover with the second slice of bread.
  - Cut in half and serve.

- **Health Benefits**:

Peanut butter offers protein and healthy fats, while bananas add natural sweetness and potassium. Whole-grain bread provides extra fiber and nutrients.

3. HUMMUS AND VEGGIE SANDWICH

- **Ingredients**:
  - 2 slices of whole-grain bread
  - 1/4 cup hummus
  - 1/4 cucumber (sliced)
  - 1/4 red bell pepper (sliced)
  - A handful of spinach leaves.

- **Preparation**:
  - Spread hummus on one slice of bread.
  - Layer cucumber, bell pepper, and spinach on top, and cover with the second slice of bread.
  - Cut in half and serve.

- Health Benefits:

Hummus is rich in protein and healthy fats. Vegetables like cucumber, bell pepper, and spinach provide essential vitamins, minerals, and fiber.

4. TURKEY AND AVOCADO SANDWICH

- Ingredients:

- 2 slices of whole-grain bread
- 2 slices of turkey breast
- 1/2 avocado (sliced)
- A handful of arugula
- mustard, or mayo (optional).

- Preparation:

- Spread mustard or mayo on one slice of bread if desired.
- Layer turkey, avocado slices, and arugula.
- Top with the second slice of bread.
- Cut in half and serve.

- Health Benefits:

Turkey provides lean protein, while avocado adds healthy fats. Arugula offers vitamins and a slight peppery taste, enhancing the flavor and nutrition of the sandwich.

5. EGG AND SPINACH BREAKFAST SANDWICH

- **Ingredients**:
  - 1 whole-grain English muffin
  - 1 egg, a handful of spinach leaves
  - 1 slice of cheese
  - Salt and pepper to taste
  - Olive oil.

- **Preparation**:
  - Toast the English muffin.
  - Heat olive oil in a skillet over medium heat and cook the egg to your liking.
  - Layer spinach leaves and cheese on the bottom half of

the muffin, place the cooked egg on top, and season with salt and pepper.

- Cover with the top half of the muffin.
- Serve immediately.

- Health Benefits:

Eggs are an excellent source of protein, while spinach provides iron and other essential nutrients. The whole-grain English muffin adds fiber, making this a well-balanced breakfast option.

Toast and sandwich combinations are practical choices for busy mornings. These recipes are designed to provide a mix of nutrients, ensuring you start your day with a wholesome meal that supports your weight loss goals.

CHAPTER 6

FRESH FRUIT AND YOGURT BOWLS

Combining fresh fruit with yogurt creates a delicious and healthy breakfast option that's quick to prepare. This chapter presents a variety of refreshing fruit and yogurt bowls, perfect for energizing your morning while supporting weight loss.

1. BERRY BLISS YOGURT BOWL

- **Ingredients**:
  - 1 cup Greek yogurt
  - 1/2 cup mixed berries (strawberries, blueberries, raspberries)
  - 1 tablespoon chia seeds
  - 1 teaspoon honey.

- **Preparation**:
  - Transfer Greek yogurt into a bowl using a spoon.
  - Top with mixed berries and sprinkle chia seeds over the top.
  - Drizzle with honey.
  - Serve immediately.

- **Health Benefits**:
Greek yogurt is rich in protein and probiotics, aiding in digestion and satiety. Berries provide antioxidants, vitamins, and fiber, while chia seeds add omega-3 fatty acids and additional fiber.

2. TROPICAL PARADISE YOGURT BOWL

- **Ingredients**:
  - 1 cup coconut yogurt
  - 1/2 cup pineapple chunks
  - 1/2 banana (sliced)
  - 1 tablespoon shredded coconut
  - 1 teaspoon flax seeds.

- **Preparation**:
  - Place coconut yogurt in a bowl.
  - Add pineapple chunks and banana slices.
  - Sprinkle shredded coconut and flax seeds on top.
  - Serve immediately.

- **Health Benefits**:

Coconut yogurt offers a dairy-free option with healthy fats, while pineapple and banana add natural sweetness and a variety of vitamins. Flax seeds provide fiber and omega-3 fatty acids.

3. PEACH AND ALMOND YOGURT BOWL

- Ingredients:

- 1 cup vanilla yogurt
- 1 fresh peach (sliced)
- 1 tablespoon sliced almonds
- 1 teaspoon honey.

- Preparation:

- Spoon vanilla yogurt into a bowl.
- Top with peach slices and sprinkle sliced almonds over the top.
- Drizzle with honey.
- Serve immediately.

- **Health Benefits**:
Vanilla yogurt provides protein and calcium. Peaches are a good source of vitamins A and C, while almonds add healthy fats and a satisfying crunch.

4. KIWI AND STRAWBERRY YOGURT BOWL

- **Ingredients**:
  - 1 cup plain yogurt
  - 1 kiwi (peeled and sliced)
  - 1/2 cup strawberries (sliced)
  - 1 tablespoon sunflower seeds
  - 1 teaspoon agave nectar.

- **Preparation**:
  - Place plain yogurt in a bowl.
  - Add kiwi and strawberry slices.
  - Sprinkle sunflower seeds on top and drizzle with agave nectar.
  - Serve immediately.

- **Health Benefits**:
Plain yogurt is a great source of protein and probiotics. Kiwi and strawberries provide a boost of vitamin C and fiber, while sunflower seeds add healthy fats and protein.

5. MANGO AND COCONUT YOGURT BOWL

- **Ingredients**:
  - 1 cup Greek yogurt
  - 1/2 cup mango chunks
  - 1 tablespoon shredded coconut
  - 1 teaspoon chia seeds.

- **Preparation**:
  - Transfer Greek yogurt into a bowl using a spoon.
  - Top with mango chunks, shredded coconut, and chia seeds.
  - Serve immediately.

- **Health Benefits**:
Greek yogurt offers high protein content and probiotics. Mango adds a tropical flavor along with vitamins A and C. Shredded coconut provides healthy fats, and chia seeds add fiber and omega-3 fatty acids.

Fruit and yogurt bowls are an excellent choice for a quick and nutritious breakfast. These recipes offer a combination of protein, healthy fats, and natural sugars to keep you satisfied and energized throughout the morning, making them a valuable addition to your weight loss plan.

CHAPTER 7

ON-THE-GO BREAKFAST SOLUTIONS

For those hectic mornings when you need a quick and portable breakfast, this chapter offers a variety of healthy and convenient recipes. These on-the-go solutions are designed to provide balanced nutrition, making it easier to stick to your weight loss goals even on the busiest days.

1. OVERNIGHT OATS IN A JAR

- **Ingredients**:
  - 1/2 cup rolled oats
  - 1/2 cup almond milk
  - 1/4 cup Greek yogurt
  - 1 tablespoon chia seeds
  - 1/2 cup mixed berries
  - 1 teaspoon honey.

- **Preparation**:
  - In a mason jar, combine rolled oats, almond milk, Greek yogurt, and chia seeds.
  - Stir well, then top with mixed berries and honey.
  - Seal the jar and refrigerate overnight.

- Grab and go in the morning.

- Health Benefits:
This easy meal provides fiber from the oats and chia seeds, protein from the yogurt, and antioxidants from the berries, making it a balanced and nutritious choice.

2. VEGGIE-PACKED EGG MUFFINS

- **Ingredients**:
  - 6 eggs, 1/2 cup spinach (chopped)
  - 1/4 cup bell peppers (diced)
  - 1/4 cup onions (diced)
  - Salt and pepper to taste
  - Olive oil.

- **Preparation**:
  - Preheat the oven to 350°F (175°C).
  - In a bowl, beat the eggs and mix in chopped spinach, bell peppers, onions, salt, and pepper.

- Grease a muffin tin with olive oil and pour the egg mixture into each cup, filling them about 3/4 full.
- Bake for 20-25 minutes or until the muffins are set.
- Let them cool, then store in the fridge for a quick breakfast throughout the week.

- Health Benefits:

These egg muffins are rich in protein and packed with vegetables, providing essential vitamins and minerals. They are a great way to start the day with a nutrient-dense meal.

3. PEANUT BUTTER BANANA WRAP

- **Ingredients**:
  - 1 whole-grain tortilla
  - 2 tablespoons peanut butter
  - 1 banana
  - 1 teaspoon honey
  - A sprinkle of cinnamon.

- **Preparation**:
  - Spread peanut butter evenly over the tortilla.
  - Place the banana in the center, drizzle with honey, and sprinkle with cinnamon.
  - Roll up the tortilla tightly and wrap it in foil for a portable breakfast.

- **Health Benefits**:
This wrap offers a good balance of protein and healthy fats from the peanut butter, natural sugars from the banana, and fiber from the whole-grain tortilla, making it a satisfying and energizing option.

4. YOGURT AND GRANOLA PARFAIT

Ingredients:
- 1 cup of Greek yogurt
- 1/2 cup of granola
- 1/2 cup of mixed berries and 1 tablespoon of honey.

- **Preparation**:
- In a portable container, layer Greek yogurt, granola, and mixed berries.
- Drizzle with honey and cover with a lid.
- Keep it refrigerated until willing to consume it.

- Health Benefits:

Greek yogurt provides protein and probiotics, granola adds fiber and crunch, and berries contribute vitamins and antioxidants, creating a well-rounded breakfast that's easy to take on the go.

5. SMOOTHIE PACKS

- Ingredients:
- 1 banana
- 1/2 cup berries
- 1/2 cup spinach
- 1 tablespoon chia seeds
- 1 cup almond milk (to add when blending).

- Preparation:
- Prepare individual smoothie packs by placing bananas, berries, spinach, and chia seeds in freezer bags.
- Store in the freezer.
- When ready to make a smoothie, pour the contents of one bag into a blender, add

almond milk, and blend until smooth.

- Transfer the contents into a portable container and savor the beverage.

- Health Benefits:

Smoothie packs offer a convenient way to enjoy a nutritious breakfast. They provide a mix of fruits, vegetables, fiber, and protein, supporting your health and weight loss efforts while saving time.

On-the-go breakfasts can help you maintain a healthy eating routine even when time is tight. These recipes ensure you have access to nutritious options that are quick, easy, and portable, allowing you to stay on track with your weight loss journey.

CONCLUSION

TIPS FOR EFFECTIVE WEIGHT LOSS

Reaching and maintaining a healthy weight involves more than just changing what you eat. It requires a comprehensive approach that integrates different aspects of your lifestyle. Here are some practical tips to support you on your weight loss journey:

1. HYDRATE PROPERLY

- Drinking enough water is essential for your body's functions and can help you manage your weight. Staying hydrated keeps you feeling full and supports your metabolism.

2. EAT MINDFULLY

- Focus on your meals without distractions. Pay attention to your hunger and fullness signals, and take your time to enjoy each bite. This can help you avoid overeating and appreciate your food more.

3. PRIORITIZE SLEEP

- Getting enough sleep is essential for managing one's weight. Aim for 7-9 hours of restful sleep each night to help regulate your metabolism and reduce cravings for unhealthy foods.

4. STAY ACTIVE

- Regular exercising is essential for a healthy lifestyle. Find activities you enjoy, such as walking, cycling, swimming, or yoga, and aim for at least 150 minutes of moderate exercise each week.

5. PLAN YOUR MEALS

- Planning and preparing your meals ahead of time can help you make healthier choices and avoid last-minute temptations. Consider batch cooking and keeping healthy snacks readily available.

6. MANAGE STRESS

- High amounts of stress can trigger emotional eating and weight gain. Practice stress-relief techniques like deep breathing, meditation, or spending time outdoors to keep stress under control.

7. KEEP A FOOD DIARY

- Writing down what you eat can help you stay accountable and notice patterns in your eating habits. Use a notebook or an app to track your meals, snacks, and drinks.

8. SET ACHIEVABLE GOALS

- Aim for realistic and attainable weight loss goals. Focus on small, sustainable changes rather than drastic shifts, and celebrate each milestone you reach along the way.

9. BUILD A SUPPORT SYSTEM

- Surround yourself with encouraging friends and family, or consider joining a weight loss club. Having a network of people who encourage you can provide motivation and accountability.

10. Reward Yourself

- Recognize your progress and reward yourself with non-food treats. Whether it's a new book, a spa day, or a fun outing, celebrating your achievements can keep you motivated.

Effective weight loss is about making lasting changes that enhance your health and happiness. By incorporating these tips into your daily routine, you can achieve your weight loss goals and maintain a balanced, healthy lifestyle.